ADE LANE

DIY Affordable Skincare v2

Combat Aging, Breakouts, and Pigmentation with Practical Skincare Solutions – No Expensive Salons Necessary!

This book was professionally typeset on Reedsy.
Find out more at reedsy.com

Contents

Foreword

Discover the secrets to radiant, youthful skin without breaking the bank. Have you ever marveled at the flawless complexion of celebrities and wondered how they maintain their beauty? Well, you'll be surprised to learn that achieving healthy, glowing skin doesn't require a hefty investment.

In this book, I share my discoveries on how I achieved rejuvenated skin at 55. After seeing a shocking photo of myself, I realized the toll of my past habits - smoking, drinking, and excessive tanning had taken on my complexion. Determined to make a change, I delved into the world of home beauty solutions. Through experimentation, training in formulation, skin peels and other treatments, I witnessed a remarkable transformation in my skin.

Geared towards those with limited time and resources, this book offers practical, affordable advice for achieving your skincare goals. You'll find simple, budget-friendly strategies that anyone can implement. Let "DIY Affordable Skincare" be your guide to a more radiant future.

1

Introduction

Understanding why our skin ages is crucial to slowing down the process. Our skin isn't just a superficial layer; it's our body's largest organ, a true multi-tasker responsible for shielding us from harm, regulating temperature, and ensuring our vital systems run smoothly. With its three main layers - the epidermis, dermis, and hypodermis constantly renewing themselves, shedding old cells and welcoming new ones at a rate of about 500 a day, it's evident that our skin craves some serious tender loving care.

However, lurking in the background is our skin's archenemy: the sun. When those harmful UV rays penetrate unprotected skin, they wreak havoc at a cellular level, causing photodamage deep within the dermis. The frightening part? It can take years for this damage to manifest visibly. That's why sunscreen is our skin's best ally. Choosing an SPF 30 or higher sunscreen, preferably labeled "broad-spectrum" to shield against both UVA and UVB rays, can truly transform our skin's aging journey over the years. Use it daily when leaving home. Personally, I swear by SPF 50, on my face, neck and chest, especially under intense sunlight, and I make it a rule never to expose my skin to its rays for more than 15 minutes at a stretch.

It's important to be aware of what goes into the skincare products we buy. When you pick up a skincare product from a store in the US, Canada, or Europe, you'll find a full rundown of its ingredients right there on the packaging. In the US, whether it's whipped up locally or shipped from afar, cosmetics have to toe the line set by the Federal Food, Drug, and Cosmetic (FD&C) Act, as well as the Fair Packaging and Labeling (FP&L) Act. But here's the kicker: those adorable homemade finds you snag at fairs or markets might not be as forthcoming about what's inside.

When you give that label a once-over, you might spot plant ingredients listed with their unfamiliar Latin names (two words) followed by their everyday names in brackets such as Lavandula angustifolia (lavender) oil and Persea Gratissima (avocado) oil.

Now, some of those ingredients might sound like they were cooked up in a lab, and there's this myth floating around that if you can't pronounce it, it's probably not good for you but that's not always true. Plenty of common or naturally derived ingredients sport long, complicated names but are perfectly safe for your skin. Check out a few examples:

- Tocopherol: Just a fancy term for vitamin E, keeping your product fresh as a daisy.
- Xanthan gum: This naturally derived gum adds some heft to your goo.
- Cetyl alcohol: This fatty alcohol is a champ at stabilizing emulsions and keeping skin hydrated.
- Citric acid: Balances the pH levels and keeps the nasties at bay.
- Sorbitan olivate: This emulsifier is simply a mix of sorbitol and olive oil.
- Potassium sorbate: A preservative made from natural sorbic acid salt, ensuring your skincare stays fresher for longer.

Safety always comes first.

If you're pregnant or currently on prescription medication, it's crucial to consult your doctor before diving into treatments involving Retinoids, Peels, and Derma rollers.

When it comes to purchasing skincare products, stick with reputable companies, and be vigilant. If you experience any adverse reactions, halt usage immediately. My hope is that you will use this book as an introduction into home skin care and follow it up with more intense training and research the vast array of information that is out there.

For your convenience, I've included a list of trusted suppliers I've used at the end of this book.

While I sing the praises of various products and treatments throughout these pages, it's essential to remember that what we put into our bodies matters just as much. As delving into that topic could fill a book of its own, I'll simply advise keeping alcohol, sugar, wheat, dairy and processed foods to a minimum. Opt for organic fruits and vegetables whenever possible, and stay hydrated by drinking plenty of filtered water - consider carrying a bottle with you whenever you're out and about. And let's not forget the dangers of smoking and tanning beds, both of which can wreak havoc on your skin - I speak from personal experience.

2

Let's Formulate

Ok - are you ready? Let's dive into the world of DIY skincare! After completing several formulation courses, I've transitioned away from store-bought products and mostly whip up my own creations. Today, I'm thrilled to share a simple moisturizer recipe with you - one that you can customize to your heart's content. Feel free to swap out oils, add your favorite essential oils for fragrance, and make it truly your own.

Formulating skincare is all about the chemical process, so paying attention to temperatures is key! Invest in a budget-friendly thermometer from Amazon to ensure precision. Once you give this recipe a shot, you won't look back! I highly recommend Aromantic.co.uk, based in the U.K. for many of the formulation ingredients and their training, but there are many others (see product Sources in Afterword).

A simple recipe for face moisturizer 100ml

    1st fat stage (75°- 80°C)

    7ml Avocado Nut Oil

    4ml Apricot Kernal Oil

8ml Baobab Oil

3g VE emulsifier

2g Cetyl Alcohol

2nd water stage (75°- 80°C)

38ml Spring Water

22ml Frankincense water

3ml Glycerine

5g MF emulsifier

3rd Stage (35°- 40°C)

1ml Preservative Eco

1ml Vitamin E Oil

4th Stage (25°- 30°-C)

Essential Oil – Rose, Frankincense or your favourite – 5-6 drops

Instructions:

1. Heat the Stage 1 (fat stage) ingredients in a double boiler until melted and @ 75°-80° C.
2. Mix the Stage 2 (water stage) ingredients together to make a slurry, then add boiling spring water @ 75°-80° C. Stick blend briefly.
3. Add the Stage 1 mixture to the Stage 2 mixture and stir thoroughly to combine the ingredients then stick blend for about 30 seconds until emulsified. It is important to stir the stages together before using the stick blender. Stop stick blending and remove from the heat.
4. Allow to cool naturally whilst stirring with a spoon or spatula continuously. Do not accelerate the cooling time in a cold-water

bath.

5. When the cream is below 40°C, add the Stage 3 ingredients and stir thoroughly, then jar and date label.

Or, if you're looking for a shortcut, here's a little hack for you! Simply grab a budget-friendly jar of skin cream and jazz it up by adding a few key "actives" - about 2-3% of each is plenty. You can mix in 2-3 different actives to elevate your cream game. For example, I've experimented with adding Niacinamide, Matrixyl, Argireline, Copper Peptides, and Hyaluronic Acid (check out Chapter 5 for more details). Brands like The Ordinary and formulation companies like Aromantic.co.uk offer a wide array of potent actives perfect for this kind of DIY upgrade – see the list of suppliers at the end of the book.

Face packs

Why not whip up your budget-friendly face packs using ingredients you likely already have in your fridge and pantry? Here are some simple ideas tailored for different skin types to get you started.

Nourishing Honey Avocado Mask (Dry Skin):
Ingredients:
1/2 ripe avocado
1 tablespoon honey
1 tablespoon plain yogurt
Instructions:

1. Mash the avocado until smooth.
2. Mix in honey and yogurt until well combined.
3. Apply the mixture to clean, dry skin and leave on for 15-20 minutes.
4. Rinse off with warm water and pat dry. Follow up with your regular

moisturizer.

Benefits: Avocado provides deep hydration and nourishment, honey soothes and moisturizes, while yogurt gently exfoliates and brightens dull skin.

Clarifying Green Tea Matcha Mask (Oily/Combination Skin):
  Ingredients:
  1 teaspoon matcha green tea powder
  1 tablespoon plain Greek yogurt
  1 teaspoon honey (optional)
  Instructions:

1. Mix matcha powder and yogurt (and honey, if using) until you get a smooth paste.
2. Apply the mixture evenly to clean skin, focusing on oily areas.
3. Leave it on for 10–15 minutes.
4. Rinse off with lukewarm water and pat dry. Follow up with oil-free moisturizer.

Benefits: Matcha green tea is rich in antioxidants and helps control oil production, yogurt gently exfoliates and balances the skin's pH, while honey adds antibacterial properties.

Soothing Oatmeal and Chamomile Mask (Sensitive Skin):
  Ingredients:
  2 tablespoons finely ground oats
  1 tablespoon chamomile tea (cooled)
  1 tablespoon plain yogurt (optional)
  Instructions:

1. Mix ground oats and chamomile tea (and yogurt, if desired) to form a thick paste.
2. Apply the mixture to clean skin, avoiding the eye area.
3. Relax for 10-15 minutes.
4. Gently rinse off with cool water and pat dry. Follow with a gentle moisturizer.

Benefits: Oats have anti-inflammatory properties to calm sensitive skin, chamomile soothes irritation and redness, while yogurt adds moisture and probiotics for a healthy skin barrier.

Brightening Turmeric and Lemon Mask (Dull/Uneven Skin Tone):
Ingredients:
1 teaspoon turmeric powder
1 tablespoon plain yogurt or milk
1 teaspoon lemon juice
Instructions:

1. Mix turmeric powder, yogurt (or milk), and lemon juice until well combined.
2. Apply the mixture evenly to clean skin, avoiding the eye area.
3. Leave it on for 10-15 minutes.
4. Rinse off with lukewarm water, gently massaging in circular motions to exfoliate, then pat dry. Follow with moisturizer and sunscreen (as lemon juice can make skin photosensitive).

Benefits: Turmeric brightens and evens out skin tone, lemon juice provides vitamin C for a radiant glow, and yogurt/milk gently exfoliates and moisturizes.

3

Vitamin C

Vitamin C is among my cherished skincare essentials, being the first product I ever formulated myself. Renowned for its ability to shield against free radical damage as an antioxidant, even out skin tone as it inhibits melanin formation, brightening and stimulate collagen synthesis, it's a cornerstone of my routine. I don't mean the Vitamin C supplement you take internally, although they are a health hit if you don't get enough in your diet and also beneficial to your skin.

You can buy topical Vitamin C liquid or serum which is usually made from L-ascorbic acid as it's the most potent, with a strength of 10% to 20% and a pH lower than 3.5. Vitamin C topical shop-bought products often have ferulic acid and Vitamin E added, enhancing their efficacy by safeguarding against environmental aggressors. **Do not** use lemon juice or straight Ascorbic acid on your skin, it's way too strong and can cause damage.

Here are a few examples of other forms of topical Vitamin C found in shop products:

- Magnesium ascorbyl phosphate (MAP) is a water-soluble form of vitamin C which converts to ascorbic acid when applied to the skin. It is very popular and used in some of the big brands C serums.

- Sodium ascorbyl phosphate - water-soluble form of vitamin C. It tends to be gentler on the skin compared to L-ascorbic acid and it is more stable.
- Sodium ascorbate - water-soluble form of vitamin C. It's a sodium salt made by replacing the 3-hydroxy group of ascorbic acid with a sodium ion. It is gentler on sensitive skin compared to L-ascorbic acid but is also less effective.
- Calcium ascorbate (CAAS) is a mineral salt of ascorbic acid and is again more stable than ascorbic acid, but it's also less potent.

However, it's worth noting that Vitamin C may not be suitable for extremely sensitive or oily skin types. My experiences with various Vitamin C products, found in a liquid or serum form, mostly sourced from Amazon at around $15, have found them to be on par with pricier counterparts from renowned brands costing up to $99. And if you get the formulation bug – make your own!

For optimal results, incorporate Vitamin C into your daily morning routine post-cleansing, by wiping it over your skin, complemented by a minimum SPF 30 sunscreen and moisturizer application after a few minutes to allow time for the Vitamin C to penetrate. To prevent potential skin irritation, avoid pairing it with other acids, particularly when used daily. Furthermore, refrain from combining it with retinol, as this can compromise its stability and hinder skin penetration. I use retinol at night before bed and Vitamin C serum in the morning and that's fine for me. If you encounter sensitivity, use Retinoids and Vitamin C on alternate days, drop one and just use the other for a couple of months. I only use Retinoids in the colder months as they are very sensitive to sunlight.

Proper storage is paramount: Vitamin C should be stored in a nontransparent glass container, shielded from direct sunlight. Fresh Vitamin C appears clear, with a slight white tint. If the solution darkens to a deep orange hue or develops a pungent odor, it has likely oxidized and should be discarded.

4

Retinoids

Retinoids, often referred to as Retin-A, constitute a group of compounds derived from vitamin A, acclaimed for their profound benefits in skincare. These retinoids encompass various types, each characterized by distinct properties and applications. Let's delve into the diverse spectrum of Retin-A derivatives and their roles in skincare to help you understand:

Retinol: Among the most widely utilized forms of retinoids in skincare, retinol serves as a milder derivative of vitamin A. Once absorbed into the skin, it undergoes conversion into retinoic acid, the active form of vitamin A. Renowned for its capacity to stimulate collagen synthesis, augment skin cell turnover, and enhance texture and tone, retinol finds extensive use in over-the-counter skincare products. It is particularly suited for individuals with sensitive skin or those venturing into retinoid usage for the first time.

Retinaldehyde: Positioned as a more potent variant of retinoid than retinol, retinaldehyde maintains a gentler profile compared to prescription-strength counterparts. Requiring one less conversion step to attain retinoic acid status, it exhibits heightened efficacy in fostering collagen production and mitigating the appearance of wrinkles and fine lines. Retinaldehyde is a prevalent component in anti-aging skincare formulations, offering visible results with diminished irritation compared to prescription retinoids.

Adapalene: A synthetic retinoid, adapalene finds widespread application in the management of acne and associated skin conditions. It impedes acne formation, inflammation reduction, and pore unclogging. Available both over-the-counter and via prescription, adapalene caters primarily to oily and acne-prone skin types, contributing to an improvement in overall skin texture and tone.

Tretinoin (Retinoic Acid): Representing the active form of vitamin A, tretinoin stands as the most potent retinoid applicable in skincare. Operating through binding to retinoic acid receptors within the skin, it elicits collagen synthesis, accelerates cell turnover, and diminishes the visibility of wrinkles, hyperpigmentation, and acne. Solely accessible via prescription, tretinoin epitomizes the pinnacle of anti-aging and acne treatment, albeit often accompanied by substantial skin irritation and sensitivity, especially during initial usage. Its efficacy in enhancing skin health and appearance remains unequivocal.

Isotretinoin (Accutane): An oral retinoid medication, isotretinoin is designated for the treatment of severe cystic acne resistant to other therapies. By curbing sebum production, averting acne lesion formation, and shrinking skin oil glands, isotretinoin exerts potent anti-acne effects. Despite its efficacy, isotretinoin carries the potential for serious side effects, including birth defects, depression, and liver impairment, warranting short-term usage under stringent medical supervision.

In summary, retinoids, encompassing a spectrum of Retin-A formulations, emerge as potent vitamin A derivatives offering multifaceted benefits for skincare. Ranging from wrinkle reduction and hyperpigmentation mitigation to acne treatment and skin texture refinement, retinoids serve as versatile components adept at addressing diverse skincare concerns. Whether integrated into over-the-counter regimes or prescribed by dermatologists, the inclusion of retinoids in skincare routines facilitates the attainment of healthier, more youthful skin.

These products are suitable for daily use, ideally applied before bedtime. A small, pea-sized amount is enough to cover the entire face, ensuring to steer clear of the delicate eye area. I find it most effective to incorporate them into my skincare routine seasonally, typically from September to April, as a precaution against the stronger sunlight during the UK summer months. However, it's crucial to adhere to the provided instructions and factor in the sun's intensity specific to your geographical location. Sun exposure while using retinoids can lead to an increase in melanin production, so it's important to exercise caution and adjust usage accordingly.

Important - It's imperative to apply a daily SPF 30 minimum sunscreen while utilizing retinoids and avoid use with Vitamin C or other acids.

5

Chemical Peels

hemical peels are a big part of my skincare routine, a journey in which I've gradually adjusted the strength and now enjoy layering two different types - Jessner and TCA - yielding noticeable salon-like results. Patience truly pays dividends – don't rush it!.

A chemical peel involves the application of acid to remove outer skin layers, stimulating new cell growth and enhancing texture and appearance while addressing specific skin concerns. The acid penetrates the epidermis in a controlled manner, offering either quick exfoliation or deeper correction of various skin issues.

Chemical peels are versatile, suitable for the face, neck, or hands, offering benefits such as reducing fine lines, treating sun-damaged wrinkles, improving mild scars, addressing acne, and diminishing age spots and dark patches. Additionally, they deeply exfoliate and brighten the skin, resulting in an overall improved look and feel, especially beneficial for sun-damaged skin.

After undergoing a chemical peel, the skin becomes temporarily more sensitive to the sun, necessitating daily sunscreen application, sun exposure limitation, and the use of wide-brimmed hats when outdoors, particularly between 10 a.m. and 2 p.m, depending on the strength of the sun in your area. While chemical peels are generally more effective on fair skin tones, individuals with darker skin can benefit provided they undergo pre-testing and adhere strictly to recommendations tailored for their skin type.

It's essential to exercise caution, especially when administering chemical peels at home, as they are more potent than over-the-counter chemical exfoliants. Gradually increasing acid strength while closely monitoring skin reactions is advised. Some popular home peel options include:

Lactic Acid

Derived from milk, lactic acid belongs to the alpha-hydroxy acids (AHAs) group. Available in varying strengths, it offers gentle exfoliation suitable for beginners. It is also available as a medium peel at 10 - 15%, and the deeper (professional) peels have even higher concentrations.

Mandelic Acid

Another AHA, the mandelic peel is a terrific choice for beginners because it's also a superficial peel. It's great at enhancing the appearance, especially of aging skin. It is not recommended for persons with rosacea or darker skin pigmentation due to its sensitive nature. It is usually available in 22% and 40% strength.

Glycolic Acid

Glycolic acid, also AHA, is derived from sugar cane and is of low molecular weight, which enables it to penetrate the skin at a deeper level. The benefits are numerous and include deep exfoliation, skin brightening, increased moisture retention and skin cell turnover. Always start with 30%.

30% - Ideal for beginners, this strength gently introduces your skin to the rejuvenating power of glycolic acid.

50% - For those familiar with chemical peels and seeking a moderate boost in their skincare regime.

70% – The most potent strength we offer, perfect for seasoned users aiming for intensive results.

Salicylic Acid

Salicylic is a beta hydroxy acid (BHA) and is designed to transform open pores and acne-prone skin. It is well-tolerated by most skin types. Following treatment, you will experience a light sloughing to deep-sheets of peeling, which will reveal soft, smooth, and revitalised skin beneath. Do not use a salicylic peel if you are pregnant.

3% – Pre-Teens, Teens and Adults multiple times per week.

15% – Weekly peel for all non-sensitive, clogged pores.

25% – Move onto once skin has fully-adjusted.

Jessner

The Jessner peel is a medium-strength peel that can be used on almost any skin type, but always skin test. It is a cocktail of various acids – usually Salicylic, Lactic and Resorcinol. It is especially beneficial for those with oily or spot-prone skin because it reduces oil production. It is recommended that this be used by the more experienced home user and used once a month initially.

TCA

A TCA peel, or Trichloroacetic Acid Peel, is a medium-strength peel that can be used to treat a variety of skin disorders. A much stronger version can only be performed at a dermatology clinic. A TCA peel can help lighten and even out skin texture and change and correct skin pigmentation. Allow a week for the healing process after a TCA peel because your skin will peel physically. It is recommended that this be used for the more experienced home user. Available in 7,13,20 & 30% strengths – start on the lowest and gradually increase.

When applying a peel, ensure to cleanse the skin, use a pre-peel solution, apply the chemical solution with caution using a fan brush or piece of gauze, squeezed out, avoiding the eyes and mouth area. Most peels are left on between 3-5 minutes, then followed up with a neutralizer or water rinse, if required. Using a peel can cause a stinging sensation, if it is too intense, or you experience excess redness then neutralize immediately with a recommended neutralizer or water.

With experience and skin adaptation, layering the same or different acids can enhance results, offering a cost-effective alternative to salon treatments.

While this overview provides merely a glimpse into the world of at-home chemical peels, thorough training and guidance, such as that offered by Platinum Skincare, are highly recommended for the safe and effective usage of these products, I took a professional skin peel course and follow Platinum for their specific information and clear advice on the different peels. Their training resources and products are highly endorsed - https://peeluniversity.com/getting-started/start-here and I can also recommend their products (see Product Resources).

6

Actives

Incorporating "actives" into your skincare routine can certainly improve elements of skin texture, tone, and overall health. Their diverse mechanisms address various skincare concerns, from combating signs of aging to enhancing skin resilience against environmental stressors. An active ingredient used in skin care has been researched and tested in a laboratory to change the skin in some way – it is active in treating something e.g. acne or dehydration.

Actives that can be added to your homemade or bought creams or serums – add 2-3% to 100 ml. cream.

Let's look at some of my favorites from the peptide family and some of the more popular actives like Hyaluronic Acid and Niacinamide.

Peptides

Peptides, are essentially smaller versions of proteins, offering multi-faceted benefits in skincare. They are recognized for their potential to provide pro-aging support, alleviate inflammation, diminish wrinkles, enhance skin firmness, and bolster blood circulation. Recent research highlights certain peptides' promising role in retarding the aging process, quelling inflammation, and combating microbial activity.

Moreover, peptides exhibit the capacity to stimulate melanin production, the skin pigment responsible for shielding against sun damage, thereby supporting the skin's natural defense.

Among the array of peptides, three stand out as personal favorites, which I integrate into my daily skincare regimen by adding 2-3% to creams:

Matrixyl®: Extensive studies conducted by researchers at the University of Reading have highlighted the efficacy of Matrixyl® in bolstering collagen levels. Results indicate that Matrixyl® can nearly double collagen production within skin cells, provided the concentration reaches optimal levels.

Argireline: Renowned for its ability to impede muscle movement associated with wrinkle formation, Argireline also demonstrates potential in promoting collagen synthesis. By optimizing collagen function, it effectively reduces fine lines and enhances skin moisture levels.

Copper Peptides: This peptide variant not only stimulates collagen production but also combats free radical damage and hyperpigmentation. Additionally, it serves as a cleansing agent, eliminating damaged collagen and elastin from the skin, thereby rejuvenating its appearance.

Hyaluronic Acid

Hyaluronic acid, often touted as the "fountain of youth" in skincare, is a naturally occurring substance in the human body, particularly abundant in connective tissues, eyes, and skin. Renowned for its exceptional ability to retain moisture, hyaluronic acid plays a pivotal role in maintaining skin hydration, suppleness, and elasticity. In skincare, it functions as a humectant, drawing moisture from the environment into the skin, thereby plumping and hydrating the complexion. Its lightweight texture allows for rapid absorption, making it suitable for all skin types, including sensitive and acne-prone skin. Regular use of hyaluronic acid can help diminish the appearance of fine lines and wrinkles, promote a smoother and more youthful complexion, and improve overall skin texture. It is commonly found in serums, moisturizers, and masks, and is typically applied after cleansing and toning, followed by the application of heavier creams or oils to seal in the hydration.

I either mix it with my cream or just pat it on the areas on my face that are excessively dry. It can be used daily.

Niacinamide

Niacinamide, also referred to as nicotinamide, represents a water-soluble form of Vitamin B3, crucial for maintaining optimal skin health. Unlike some vitamins that the body stores, niacinamide isn't retained by the body, emphasizing the importance of replenishing it regularly. It's noteworthy that the niacinamide utilized in skincare products is entirely synthetically derived, ensuring consistency and purity. When applied topically, niacinamide exhibits remarkable versatility in its actions on the skin, readily penetrating the skin barrier and elevating levels of nicotinamide adenine dinucleotide (NAD) within skin cells.

The benefits of niacinamide in skincare are dependent upon the concentration applied, with six primary actions standing out:

- Antipruritic (Soothing): Niacinamide exerts a calming effect on the skin, alleviating itchiness and discomfort, making it particularly beneficial for sensitive or irritated skin.
- Antimicrobial (Microorganism-Killing): With its ability to combat microorganisms, niacinamide helps to maintain skin cleanliness and prevent the proliferation of acne-causing bacteria, contributing to clearer skin.
- Vasoactive (Improving Circulation): By enhancing blood circulation in the skin, niacinamide promotes a healthy complexion, aiding

in the delivery of essential nutrients and oxygen to skin cells for optimal function.

- Photoprotective (Sun Damage Protection): Acting as a shield against UV radiation, niacinamide offers protection from sun damage, helping to prevent premature aging, sunspots, and other photo-induced skin concerns.
- Sebostatic (Sebum-Reducing): Niacinamide regulates sebum production, making it an invaluable asset in managing oily or acne-prone skin, leading to a more balanced and matte complexion.
- Lightening (Dark Spot Fading): Known for its depigmenting properties, niacinamide helps fade dark spots and hyperpigmentation, promoting a more even skin tone and a radiant complexion.

Incorporating niacinamide into skincare routines can address a myriad of concerns, from soothing sensitivity to combating acne and brightening uneven skin tone. Its compatibility with various skin types and its multifaceted benefits makes it a staple ingredient in many skincare formulations.

I add 2-3% to my skin cream which can be used daily but check for sensitivity and if it appears, reduce the % of the active used in the cream or use on alternate days. You can add different actives to separate jars of cream and use them alternatively.

Derma roller

Derma rolling, also known as microneedling, is a transformative skincare practice wherein a small roller device, adorned with tiny needles, is rolled over the skin to create controlled micro-injuries in the skin. This process prompts the skin's healing mechanisms, bringing about an array of benefits, including heightened collagen production, refined skin texture, and amplified absorption of skincare products. A medical research study undertaken in 2002 with nearly 500 patients, involving the controlled disruption of the epidermis using a needle drum had remarkable results, showing a substantial 60% - 80% improvement in collagen and elastin fibres.

A range of derma rollers are available, distinguished by needle length and material composition. The epidermis is about 0.1 - 0.2 mm thick and the dermis is around 1- 2 mm thick.

Needle Length: Derma rollers span a spectrum of needle lengths, ranging from 0.25mm to 2.5mm. Shorter needles are adept at superficial exfoliation and bolstering product absorption, whereas longer needles excel in addressing deeper skin concerns like acne scars and wrinkles. I'd recommend starting with a recommended Titanium 0.25mm needle and slowly building up to 0.5mm for home use.

Needle Material: Derma roller needles are crafted from stainless steel, titanium, or medical-grade silicone. Stainless steel and titanium, renowned for their durability and efficacy, are most commonly used, while silicone needles offer a gentler approach, potentially suiting sensitive skin types.

You can use derma roller 1-2 times a week so long as any inflammation and redness has subsided. Results can be seen after a few weeks of regular use.

Benefits of Derma Rolling:

- Stimulates Collagen Production: Micro-injuries induced by derma rolling kickstart the skin's natural reparative processes, culminating in heightened collagen and elastin synthesis. This contributes to enhanced skin elasticity and firmness.
- Improves Skin Texture: Derma rolling facilitates the smoothing of uneven skin texture, diminishing the appearance of fine lines, wrinkles, and enlarged pores.
- Enhances Product Absorption: Micro-channels created during derma rolling pave the way for skincare products to permeate deeply into the skin, optimizing their efficacy and delivering superior results.
- Reduces Hyperpigmentation: Derma rolling aids in fading dark spots, acne scars, and various forms of hyperpigmentation by fostering cellular turnover and collagen remodeling.

It's advised to avoid Derma rolling if any of the following conditions apply:

- An ongoing infection in the treatment area, or if you're feeling

unwell.
- Abnormal scarring, such as keloids.
- Loose skin, particularly if treating stretch marks.
- Certain medical conditions which require prescription medication – always check.
- Allergic reactions to local anesthesia.
- Bleeding disorders or autoimmune diseases.
- Pregnancy or breastfeeding.
- Using steroid or medications that affect bleeding, like aspirin or warfarin.

How to Derma Roll:

1. Begin by cleansing your skin and disinfecting the derma roller with 70% isopropyl alcohol for a few minutes.
2. If using a topical anesthetic to numb the skin, it will normally take up to 30 minutes for it to work. Wipe a thick enough layer all over the area to be treated,
3. Use gentle, yet deliberate rolling motions in horizontal, vertical, and diagonal directions, to stroke the derma roller across the skin 2-3 times, applying light pressure.
4. Focus on one area at a time, steering clear of sensitive regions like the eyes.
5. Immediately following derma rolling, apply serums or skincare products to capitalize on heightened absorption opportunities.
6. Post-treatment, cleanse the derma roller once more and allow it to air-dry before storing it in a clean, disinfected container.

Do not use any strong acids for a few days after using a derma roller as it can cause a reaction, although products, like Vitamin C can be added to the treatment after rolling for deeper penetration. While derma rolling can be executed in the comfort of one's home, it may cause redness and mild discomfort, particularly with longer needles. Beginning treatment with shorter needles of 0.25mm and gradually advance to longer lengths as skin tolerance builds is prudent. Prior consultation with a dermatologist or skincare professional is recommended, especially for individuals with sensitive or acne-prone skin, to ensure a safe result.

It's important to recognize that rollers designed for home use typically feature shorter needle lengths and, as a result, may not yield the same benefits as microneedling procedures administered by practitioners. Ensuring both the skin and the device are thoroughly cleansed with an antiseptic solution is essential to mitigate the risk of infection.

Important - If pregnant or taking prescription medication always check with your Doctor before using a derma roller.

Afterword

I hope you have found some pointers in "DIY Affordable Skincare" which offers a quick starter guide to achieving radiant and healthy skin without breaking the bank. From DIY treatments to budget-friendly products, this book empowers the reader to take charge of their skincare routines with confidence and ease. By exploring a myriad of tips and techniques as well as affordable alternatives to salon treatments, you can embark on a journey toward glowing skin from the comfort of your own home. With practical advice and accessible solutions, "DIY Affordable Skincare" shows that achieving beautiful skin doesn't have to come with a hefty price tag. By exploring a myriad of tips and techniques, and affordable alternatives to salon treatments, you can embark on a journey toward glowing skin from the comfort of your own home.

Now you have everything you need to have beautiful skin at any age, it's time to pass on your newfound knowledge and show other readers where they can find the same help.

Simply by leaving your honest opinion of this book on Amazon in feedback, you'll show others where they can find the information they're looking for, and pass your passion for - "DIY Affordable Skincare" - forward.

Thank you for your support.

Ade

x

Resources

Nutrition, C. F. F. S. a. A. (2022, February 25). *Cosmetics Labeling Guide.* U.S. Food And Drug Administration. https://www.fda.gov/cosmetics/cosmetics-labeling-regulations/cosmetics-labeling-guide#clga

Health Canada. (2023, December 4). *Industry Guide for the labelling of cosmetics.* Canada.ca. https://www.canada.ca/en/health-canada/services/consumer-product-safety/reports-publications/industry-professionals/labelling-cosmetics.html

Cosmereg. (2023b, February 5). *EU cosmetic labeling requirements.* Cosmereg. https://cosmereg.com/eu-cosmetic-labeling-requirements

Rhue, H. (2024, February 22). 11 Best Anti-Aging Ingredients that are Clinically-Proven, according to Derms. *Byrdie.* https://www.byrdie.com/anti-aging-ingredients-biology

Cosmereg. (2023, February 5). *EU cosmetic labeling requirements.* Cosmereg. https://cosmereg.com/eu-cosmetic-labeling-requirements

Garethdespres. (2024b, March 18). *How to read a cosmetic label (the ultimate guide) -School of Natural Skincare.* School of Natural Skincare. https://www.schoolofnaturalskincare.com/how-to-read-a-cosmetic-label

Garethdespres. (2024, March 18). *How to read a cosmetic label (the ultimate guide) -School of Natural Skincare.* School of Natural Skincare. https://www.schoolofnaturalskincare.com/how-to-read-a-cosmetic-label

Home. (n.d.). PubMed Central (PMC). https://www.ncbi.nlm.nih.gov/pmc/articles/PMC10669284

Chemical peels and your skin. (2023, September 18). WebMD. https://www.webmd.com/beauty/cosmetic-procedures-chemical-peel-treatments

Paula's Choice. (n.d.). *At-home chemical face peels | Paula's Choice.*

www.paulaschoice.co.uk. https://www.paulaschoice.co.uk/at-home-chemical-face-peels

Chedik, L., Baybekov, S., Cosnier, F., Marcou, G., Varnek, A., & Champmartin, C. (2024). An update of skin permeability data based on a systematic review of recent research. *Scientific Data, 11*(1). https://doi.org/10.1038/s41597-024-03026-4

Leonard, J. (2023, August 16). *What to know about peptides for health.* https://www.medicalnewstoday.com/articles/326701#how-to-use

Microneedling. (n.d.). BCAM. https://bcam.ac.uk/patients/treatments/microneedling.aspx

Product Sources

- https://aromantic.co.uk
- https://makingcosmetics.com
- http://naturallythinking.com
- https://theordinary.com
- https://www.platinumskincare.com
- https://www.makeupartistschoice.com
- https://www.dermaroller.com/en
- https://www.dermarollershop.com

Forums

- https://www.skincaretalk.com

www.ingramcontent.com/pod-product-compliance
Lightning Source LLC
Chambersburg PA
CBHW051723250726
48653CB00008B/3167